CW00403044

What Are White Blood Cells?

Book Chapters:

Book Introduction:

In a world teetering on the edge of chaos, where darkness threatens to engulf every soul, there exists an extraordinary force that stands as a beacon of hope. This force, hidden within the depths of every being, lies dormant, waiting to be awakened. "The Guardians Within" is a captivating journey that explores the realms of courage, resilience, and the indomitable spirit residing in each of us.

Within the pages of this book, we delve into the very essence of what it means to be human. We encounter the white blood cells—the guardians of life, tirelessly fighting against the invading forces that threaten our existence. But beyond the realm of biology, these cells symbolize something far greater—a representation of our own inner strength and determination.

Chapter 1: Awakening of the Guardians

In the quiet solitude of the human body, a silent battle rages. Unseen by the naked eye, legions of white blood cells stand ever vigilant, ready to defend their domain. In this chapter, we meet a young white blood cell named Elysia, who is about to embark on a transformative journey. Elysia possesses a unique gift—the ability to tap into the emotions of the body she inhabits.

Elysia's journey begins when she awakens to the cries of distress echoing throughout her host. Drawn by an inexplicable force, she ventures deep into the recesses of the body, guided by an instinctual desire to protect. As she traverses the complex network of blood vessels, she witnesses firsthand the ravages of an ongoing battle against a formidable enemy.

In the midst of chaos, Elysia encounters a weary red blood cell named Aiden, whose unwavering determination to keep the body alive inspires her. Together, they navigate the treacherous terrain, evading the clutches of viruses and bacteria that threaten to overpower them. Along the way, Elysia discovers that her ability to sense emotions grants her a deeper connection with the body she serves, allowing her to anticipate danger and devise strategic maneuvers.

As Elysia's powers awaken, she realizes that her purpose extends beyond merely fighting off invaders. She becomes a beacon of hope for her fellow cells, instilling courage and resilience in their weary hearts. In this chapter, we witness the birth of a hero, as Elysia embraces her destiny and prepares to face the challenges that lie ahead.

Emotional Tone:

Within the depths of "The Guardians Within," emotions run deep. From the pulsating adrenaline of a battle fought against insurmountable odds to the tender moments of camaraderie and sacrifice, the book evokes a wide range of emotions. Readers will find themselves captivated by the characters' courage, moved by their unwavering resolve, and touched by the profound connections forged amidst chaos. Through the power of storytelling, "The Guardians Within" explores the depths of the human spirit, reminding us that even in our darkest moments, we possess the strength to rise above and protect what we hold dear.

Chapter 2: Unleashing the Power Within

As Elysia continues her journey through the intricate pathways of the human body, a sense of purpose pulses within her. She senses a dormant power lingering deep within her being, waiting to be unleashed. In this chapter, we witness the transformative awakening of Elysia's true potential.

Guided by an unyielding determination, Elysia seeks out the ancient guardians of the body—the cells that hold the key to unlocking her hidden powers. These wise and experienced cells reveal the ancient wisdom passed down through generations, teaching her the secrets of her lineage.

Through rigorous training and introspection, Elysia learns to channel her emotions into a formidable force. She discovers that her tears of sorrow hold the power of healing, mending wounds and soothing the aching hearts of her fellow cells. Her laughter becomes a beacon of joy, spreading warmth and rejuvenation to those around her. And in moments of righteous anger, she ignites a blazing fire within, obliterating any threat that dares to cross her path.

But with great power comes great responsibility. Elysia grapples with the weight of her newfound abilities, understanding that their misuse could bring devastation. She learns the delicate balance between wielding strength and showing compassion, realizing that true power lies not in domination but in the service of others.

In this chapter, we witness Elysia's journey of self-discovery, as she harnesses her emotions and taps into the wellspring of power within. Her evolution is not only physical but also deeply emotional, as she learns to navigate the intricate dance between vulnerability and strength.

Emotional Tone:

Chapter 2 embraces a symphony of emotions. It unveils the raw intensity of self-discovery, as Elysia uncovers the depths of her potential. Readers will feel the surge of anticipation as Elysia embarks on her training, the awe-inspired wonder as she learns the ancient wisdom, and the tingling excitement as she begins to tap into her dormant power. The emotional landscape is rich and varied, echoing the complexities of the human experience. From the jubilant highs of newfound abilities to the poignant introspection of responsibility, the emotional tone weaves a tapestry that will resonate with readers on a profound level.

Note: Please let me know if you would like me to continue writing the subsequent chapters or if there's anything specific you would like me to focus on.

Chapter 3: The Dance of Life and Death

In the midst of the ever-changing battlefield, Elysia finds herself facing the harsh reality of life's fragility. In this chapter, emotions run deep as she witnesses the delicate dance between life and death.

As Elysia ventures deeper into the body, she encounters a group of cells engaged in a desperate struggle against a relentless virus. The battle is fierce, and the odds seem insurmountable.

Elysia's heart aches as she witnesses the sacrifice and bravery displayed by her fellow cells, who fight valiantly to protect the body they call home.

Amidst the chaos, Elysia forms a profound connection with a red blood cell named Liam. Together, they navigate the treacherous battleground, their steps guided by a shared purpose —to safeguard the fragile balance of life within. With each passing moment, the weight of their mission bears down on them, as they witness the devastating toll of the virus's relentless onslaught.

In this chapter, emotions surge to the surface as Elysia grapples with the harsh realities of mortality. She experiences the bittersweet symphony of hope and despair, love and loss. The emotional depth reaches its peak as Elysia confronts the agonizing decision to risk her own existence to save others.

Elysia learns that life is a delicate tapestry, woven with threads of resilience and vulnerability, courage and fear. The dance of life and death intertwines with her every step, reminding her of the fragility and preciousness of existence.

Emotional Tone:

Chapter 3 tugs at the heartstrings, immersing readers in a whirlwind of emotions. The raw power of love and sacrifice, the overwhelming grief of loss, and the resolute determination to protect what is dear resonate on a profoundly emotional level. Readers will find themselves teetering on the edge of their seats, gripped by the rollercoaster of emotions that permeate every . The emotional tone in this chapter encapsulates the profound complexities of life, reminding us of the beauty that can be found amidst the most challenging circumstances.

Note: Please let me know if you would like me to continue writing the subsequent chapters or if there's anything specific you would like me to focus on.

Chapter 4: Bonds that Transcend Time

In the depths of adversity, bonds are forged that defy the limitations of time and space. Chapter 4 delves into the profound connections that arise amidst the chaos and turmoil, as Elysia discovers the enduring power of unity and friendship.

As Elysia continues her relentless pursuit to protect the body, she encounters a group of cells from diverse backgrounds, each with their own unique strengths and stories. Despite their differences, a shared purpose unites them—a fervent desire to defend the fragile sanctuary they call home.

In this chapter, emotions intertwine and weave a tapestry of camaraderie and loyalty. Elysia forms deep bonds with cells from various lineages, transcending the boundaries of their individual roles. Together, they become a formidable force, their collective strength far surpassing the sum of their parts.

Through trials and tribulations, laughter and tears, these bonds deepen, creating a support network that fuels their resilience. Elysia learns that true strength lies not solely within herself but in the unwavering support and trust of her newfound companions. They lift each other up, lending a helping hand when hope wanes and celebrating victories together.

Emotional Tone:

Chapter 4 embraces the power of human connection and the emotions that arise when individuals come together for a common cause. Readers will feel a surge of warmth as the bonds of friendship are forged, and a sense of belonging as Elysia discovers her place within this extraordinary collective. The emotional tone resonates with authenticity, evoking empathy and a profound appreciation for the strength that arises when hearts unite. In this chapter, the power of unity becomes a beacon of hope, reminding readers of the transformative impact that genuine connections can have in the face of adversity.

Note: Please let me know if you would like me to continue writing the subsequent chapters or if there's anything specific you would like me to focus on.

Chapter 5: Shadows of the Past

Amidst the ceaseless battles, fragments of forgotten memories start to resurface within Elysia's consciousness. Chapter 5 delves into the haunting echoes of the past, unraveling a hidden tapestry of secrets and revelations.

As Elysia confronts a particularly menacing bacterial invasion, she finds herself drawn into the enigmatic depths of the body's history. Whispers of forgotten tales and long-lost conflicts echo through her mind, leaving a lingering sense of unease. Elysia embarks on a quest to uncover the truth, determined to shed light on the shadows that haunt the body.

With each step, Elysia unearths fragments of forgotten battles fought by her predecessors. She encounters cells whose scars bear witness to ancient struggles against formidable foes. Through their stories, she gains insight into the sacrifices made, the triumphs achieved, and the price paid to maintain the delicate equilibrium within.

But as she delves deeper into the body's history, Elysia uncovers a truth that shakes her to her core. The shadows of the past hold not only tales of heroism but also the seeds of betrayal and corruption. Loyalties are tested, and trust hangs by a fragile thread. Elysia grapples with her own role in this complex tapestry, questioning her purpose and the repercussions of the knowledge she unearths.

Emotional Tone:

Chapter 5 embraces an emotional tone filled with intrigue, suspense, and a touch of melancholy. The revelations of the past carry a weight that reverberates through the narrative, tugging at the reader's heartstrings. The emotional landscape is layered, with moments of tension, sorrow, and even a glimmer of hope. Readers will find themselves engrossed in Elysia's journey as she unravels the mysteries that lie hidden within the shadows of the body's history. In this chapter, emotions flow like an undercurrent, heightening the sense of anticipation and immersing readers in the captivating tale of forgotten truths.

Note: Please let me know if you would like me to continue writing the subsequent chapters or if there's anything specific you would like me to focus on.

Chapter 6: Embracing the Inner Light

In the wake of the revelations that have shaken her to the core, Elysia finds herself at a crossroads. Chapter 6 delves into the transformative power of self-discovery and the unwavering strength found within.

Haunted by the shadows of the past, Elysia embarks on a journey of introspection and self-reflection. She grapples with the choices that lie before her, torn between the darkness that threatens to consume and the flickering light of hope that beckons from within.

In this chapter, emotions surge as Elysia confronts her own fears and doubts. She seeks solace in the nurturing embrace of her newfound companions, drawing strength from their unwavering support. Together, they embark on a quest to uncover the source of the corruption that taints the body, determined to restore balance and harmony.

Through moments of vulnerability and resilience, Elysia discovers a wellspring of inner light within her. She learns to trust in her instincts, embracing her unique gifts, and channeling them towards the greater good. It is in the depths of her own soul that she finds the courage to face the darkness head-on, knowing that her light can pierce through even the most formidable shadows.

In this chapter, emotions run deep as Elysia's journey becomes a mirror for our own battles with self-doubt and the triumph of self-acceptance. Readers will be captivated by the raw authenticity of Elysia's transformation, feeling a surge of inspiration and hope. The emotional tone resonates with vulnerability and empowerment, reminding us that even in our darkest moments, we possess the strength to shine brightly and make a difference.

Note: Please let me know if you would like me to continue writing the subsequent chapters or if there's anything specific you would like me to focus on.

Chapter 7: Trials of Courage

As Elysia and her companions journey deeper into the heart of the body, they are faced with trials that test their courage to the limits. Chapter 7 explores the indomitable spirit that arises in the face of adversity and the profound transformations that occur through acts of bravery.

The body's inner landscape becomes treacherous, with unforeseen challenges lurking around every corner. Elysia and her companions encounter formidable viruses, each more cunning and relentless than the last. They are pushed to their physical and emotional limits, their very existence hanging in the balance.

In this chapter, emotions surge as fear intertwines with determination. Elysia's heart pounds with anticipation as she confronts her deepest anxieties, rallying her inner strength to protect those she holds dear. The bonds between her and her companions grow stronger, fortified by shared experiences of triumph and loss.

Amidst the chaos, Elysia discovers an unwavering wellspring of courage within her. She taps into reserves of resilience she never knew existed, refusing to yield even when the odds seem insurmountable. Her actions inspire her fellow cells, instilling a sense of unwavering hope and a renewed belief in their own capabilities.

Through selfless acts and unwavering resolve, Elysia and her companions emerge transformed. They find within themselves the bravery to confront their deepest fears, recognizing that true courage is not the absence of fear, but rather the willingness to face it head-on.

In this chapter, emotions soar as readers witness the awe-inspiring power of the human spirit. The courage exhibited by Elysia and her companions serves as a poignant reminder that bravery is not reserved for the extraordinary, but lies dormant within each of us. The emotional tone evokes a sense of awe, igniting a fire within readers' hearts and inspiring them to embrace their own trials with unwavering courage.

Note: Please let me know if you would like me to continue writing the subsequent chapters or if there's anything specific you would like me to focus on.

Chapter 8: Echoes of Hope

Amidst the trials and tribulations, whispers of hope echo through the body's corridors. Chapter 8 delves into the transformative power of hope and the resounding impact it has on the human spirit.

As Elysia and her companions press forward, they encounter cells and organisms fighting against the encroaching darkness with unwavering determination. Tales of resilience and triumph reverberate through the body, each one a testament to the enduring power of hope.

In this chapter, emotions swell as hope becomes a beacon of light in the midst of despair. Elysia witnesses acts of kindness, selflessness, and unwavering belief in a better tomorrow. The collective spirit of those she encounters resonates with a profound sense of optimism and possibility.

Elysia, fueled by the echoes of hope, embraces her role as a catalyst for change. She rallies her companions, inspiring them to push forward with unwavering resolve. Together, they become agents of transformation, instilling a renewed sense of purpose within the body's cells and organisms.

In the face of adversity, hope becomes an unstoppable force, infusing every step with determination and a belief in the power of the human spirit. Elysia and her companions become harbingers of hope, forging a path through the darkness and lighting the way for others to follow.

In this chapter, emotions run deep as readers experience the profound impact of hope on the human soul. The emotional tone resonates with optimism, invigorating readers' spirits and reminding them of the strength that lies within. It serves as a testament to the enduring power of hope, even in the face of overwhelming odds.

Note: Please let me know if you would like me to continue writing the subsequent chapters or if there's anything specific you would like me to focus on.

Chapter 9: In the Face of Darkness

In the heart of the body, Elysia and her companions find themselves confronting a darkness that threatens to consume all they hold dear. Chapter 9 delves into the depths of despair and the resilience that emerges when faced with the most daunting of challenges.

As they venture deeper into the body, the darkness grows more menacing. Shadows loom, and uncertainty shrouds their every step. Elysia's heart is heavy with the weight of the battle ahead, but she refuses to surrender to despair.

In this chapter, emotions intensify as the characters confront their deepest fears and doubts. Elysia grapples with moments of self-doubt, questioning her own strength and ability to overcome the encroaching darkness. Yet, within the depths of despair, a spark of resilience ignites.

Amidst the darkness, Elysia and her companions find solace in each other. They draw strength from the unyielding support they offer, reminding one another of the importance of their mission. Together, they become beacons of light in the face of overwhelming odds, refusing to let the darkness extinguish their hope.

In this chapter, emotions surge as readers are immersed in the characters' struggles. They will experience the depths of despair alongside Elysia and her companions, feeling the weight of their burdens and the relentless pressure of the darkness. Yet, within the emotional turmoil, there is an undercurrent of determination and resilience, reminding readers that even in the face of the darkest moments, the human spirit has the power to persevere.

Note: Please let me know if you would like me to continue writing the subsequent chapters or if there's anything specific you would like me to focus on.

Chapter 10: Unraveling the Secrets

In the midst of the looming darkness, Elysia and her companions stumble upon hidden secrets that hold the key to unraveling the mysteries of the body. Chapter 10 explores the emotional depths of discovery and the transformative impact of knowledge.

Driven by an unrelenting curiosity, Elysia delves into the enigmatic depths of the body's intricate systems. Clues and fragments of forgotten truths guide her path as she unravels the intricate tapestry woven within.

In this chapter, emotions intertwine as excitement mingles with trepidation. Elysia uncovers secrets that shake the very foundation of her understanding, challenging her perceptions and deepening the complexity of their mission. The weight of responsibility settles upon her shoulders as she realizes the magnitude of the knowledge she possesses.

Through the revelations, Elysia and her companions are forced to confront the true nature of the darkness that plagues the body. They find themselves grappling with the dualities of light and shadow, love and betrayal, and the fragile balance that keeps the body's existence intact.

In the face of these revelations, Elysia's resolve strengthens. She becomes a beacon of clarity amidst the confusion, guiding her companions through the labyrinth of secrets. Together, they navigate the intricacies of the body, driven by a collective determination to restore harmony and reveal the truth.

In this chapter, emotions intensify as readers are swept up in the process of unraveling the secrets. The emotional tone resonates with a blend of intrigue, awe, and uncertainty, mirroring the characters' emotional journey. It serves as a reminder of the transformative power of knowledge and the emotional impact it has on those who seek it.

Note: Please let me know if you would like me to continue writing the subsequent chapters or if there's anything specific you would like me to focus on.

Chapter 11: The Healing Touch

Amidst the revelations and the darkness that surrounds them, a glimmer of hope emerges. Chapter 11 delves into the transformative power of healing and the profound impact of compassion and empathy.

As Elysia and her companions navigate the intricacies of the body, they encounter cells and organisms ravaged by the battles that have waged within. Their hearts ache as they witness the toll of the ongoing war. But within their pain lies a calling—to bring healing to those who suffer.

In this chapter, emotions intertwine as Elysia and her companions embark on a mission of compassion. They reach out with a gentle touch, offering solace and comfort to those in need. Through their empathy and understanding, they become healers, mending not only physical wounds but also the scars that linger deep within the soul.

Elysia discovers the extraordinary power of her tears, which hold within them the essence of healing. Her tears fall like drops of pure compassion, bringing relief and renewal to the weary cells they touch. She embraces her role as a healer, channeling her emotions to soothe and uplift those she encounters.

In the midst of chaos, a sense of unity emerges. Elysia and her companions forge bonds not only with each other but also with the body itself. They become conduits of healing, offering a glimmer of hope amidst the darkness.

In this chapter, emotions swell as readers witness the profound impact of compassion and empathy. The emotional tone resonates with tenderness and warmth, evoking a deep sense of connection and reminding readers of the transformative power of a healing touch. It serves as a poignant reminder that even in the midst of turmoil, acts of kindness and understanding have the power to bring profound healing to both body and soul.

Note: Please let me know if you would like me to continue writing the subsequent chapters or if there's anything specific you would like me to focus on.

Chapter 12: Into the Abyss

As Elysia and her companions delve deeper into the body's core, they confront the abyss—the heart of darkness that threatens to consume everything in its path. Chapter 12 explores the emotional depths of despair and the unyielding spirit that emerges in the face of the unknown.

The abyss looms before them, a void that challenges their very existence. Elysia's heart quivers with a mix of fear and determination as she gazes into the depths, uncertainty clouding her thoughts. Yet, a flicker of hope burns within her, refusing to be extinguished.

In this chapter, emotions intertwine as the characters confront their deepest fears and doubts. The weight of the impending battle bears down on them, the very fabric of their courage stretched to its limits. Each step forward feels like a leap into the unknown, a choice between succumbing to the abyss or pushing through with unwavering resilience.

In the face of such darkness, Elysia and her companions draw strength from one another. They hold hands, their collective determination radiating a light that pierces through the gloom. Together, they march into the abyss, guided by an unyielding spirit that refuses to bow to despair.

In the depths of the abyss, they encounter challenges that test their resolve. The darkness seeks to dishearten and disorient, but Elysia and her companions find solace in the bonds they have forged. With every step, they discover newfound depths of courage, a resilience that emerges from the darkest corners of their souls.

In this chapter, emotions surge as readers join Elysia and her companions on their treacherous journey into the abyss. The emotional tone resonates with a mix of apprehension, determination, and a flicker of hope. It serves as a reminder that even in the face of the greatest trials, the human spirit has the capacity to shine brightly and conquer the darkest of challenges.

Note: Please let me know if you would like me to continue writing the subsequent chapters or if there's anything specific you would like me to focus on.

Chapter 13: Ripples of Change

In the heart of the abyss, Elysia and her companions confront the pivotal moment that holds the potential for immense change. Chapter 13 delves into the emotional currents that surge through their journey and the profound impact of their actions.

As they navigate the depths of darkness, Elysia and her companions come face to face with the very source of the body's affliction. The truth unfolds before them, illuminating the magnitude of the battle they must fight. Emotions churn within them—fear, anger, and a resolute determination to make a difference.

In this chapter, emotions intertwine as Elysia and her companions grapple with the weight of their choices. They are confronted by the far-reaching consequences of their actions, knowing that their decisions will send ripples through the body, shaping its future.

Together, they rally their collective strength, drawing upon the bonds they have forged and the lessons they have learned. The emotional landscape is charged with urgency as they take a stand against the forces that seek to undermine the body's well-being. Their actions reverberate with the power of determination and the unwavering belief that change is possible.

In the face of adversity, Elysia and her companions become catalysts for transformation. They challenge the status quo, sparking a revolution within the body that echoes beyond their immediate surroundings. With every step forward, they inspire others to rise, igniting a flame of resilience and hope that spreads like wildfire.

In this chapter, emotions soar as readers witness the profound impact of courageous choices. The emotional tone resonates with a mix of intensity, purpose, and a hint of apprehension. It serves as a reminder that even the smallest actions can create ripples of change, shaping the course of lives and the destiny of the body as a whole.

Note: Please let me know if you would like me to continue writing the subsequent chapters or if there's anything specific you would like me to focus on.

Chapter 14: The Ultimate Sacrifice

In the climactic chapter of their journey, Elysia and her companions face the ultimate test of their courage and commitment. Chapter 14 delves into the depths of sacrifice and the emotional resonance of selflessness.

As they stand on the precipice of a final battle, Elysia and her companions confront the daunting reality of the sacrifices they must make. Emotions swirl within them—fear, love, and an unwavering determination to protect the body they have come to know and cherish.

In this chapter, emotions intertwine as Elysia and her companions grapple with the weight of their choices. They recognize the gravity of the task at hand and the personal costs it may entail. Each decision carries the potential for immense loss, yet they find solace in the knowledge that their sacrifice is driven by a deep-seated love for the body and all it represents.

Together, they forge a pact—a solemn commitment to lay down their own well-being for the greater good. The emotional landscape is charged with a mix of sorrow and resilience as they prepare themselves for what lies ahead. They draw strength from one another, their unwavering bond a beacon in the midst of the storm.

In the face of impending battle, Elysia and her companions exemplify the true essence of selflessness. They embrace the weight of sacrifice, knowing that their actions will shape the body's destiny. Their unwavering dedication serves as a testament to the boundless capacity of love and the lengths one will go to protect what is cherished.

In this chapter, emotions reach their peak as readers witness the heart-wrenching decisions and the profound impact of selfless acts. The emotional tone resonates with a mix of sorrow, love, and unwavering resolve. It serves as a reminder that sometimes the greatest acts of heroism come from those who are willing to make the ultimate sacrifice.

Note: Please let me know if you would like me to continue writing the final chapter or if there's anything specific you would like me to focus on.

Chapter 15: Resurgence of the Guardians

In the climactic conclusion of their arduous journey, Elysia and her companions stand at the precipice of victory or defeat. Chapter 15 delves into the emotional depths of resilience and the transformative power of unity.

As the final battle unfolds, emotions surge within Elysia and her companions. Fear and determination intertwine, their hearts pounding with a mix of anticipation and trepidation. They know that this is the defining moment—the culmination of their sacrifices and unwavering commitment.

In this chapter, emotions intertwine as Elysia and her companions draw upon the depths of their courage. They unleash their collective strength, a force fueled by their shared purpose and the bonds they have forged. The emotional landscape is charged with intensity and unwavering resolve as they face the darkness with unwavering determination.

With every blow, every act of defiance, they reclaim the body from the clutches of darkness. Their resilience becomes a beacon of hope that cuts through the shadows, inspiring others to rise and join their cause. The battle rages on, but their spirit remains unyielding.

In the face of overwhelming odds, Elysia and her companions exemplify the power of unity and resilience. They embody the indomitable spirit of the guardians within, proving that even in the darkest of moments, light can prevail. Their collective strength serves as a testament to the transformative power of unity and the unwavering belief in the triumph of good over evil.

In this final chapter, emotions soar as readers witness the resurgent power of the guardians. The emotional tone resonates with a mix of triumph, relief, and a touch of bittersweetness. It serves as a reminder that even in the face of insurmountable challenges, the human spirit has the capacity to rise, overcome, and create a better future.

Note: The book has now reached its conclusion. If you have any additional requests or if there's anything specific you would like me to focus on, please let me know.